See Their Light

Empowering life lessons from those with dementia

Luminous Ones

Grandma Eileen, Auntie Melanie, Auntie Chris.
Friends, family, and all those we have been called to serve.

You are the light of the world,
a city on a hill that cannot be hidden.
Don't cover your light and hide it away.
Instead, put it on a stand for all to see.
Let it shine on everyone in the house;
a light for all who live there.

(Adapted from Matthew 5:14-15)

CONTENTS

INTRODUCTION

We work in hospice serving people with dementia. Steve is a chaplain; Marlo is a registered nurse. These are our personal notes, reflections, and stories gathered from working with some of the finest human beings we have ever met.[1]

Dementia is a very difficult disease for families to navigate. It will relentlessly chip away at years of personhood such that in the end, we are left with just a glimpse of the One we knew. Those who named their children are unable to recall them. Those who cooked family meals are unable to feed themselves. Those who have been someone's constant companion, with whom they made many memories, are now a stranger to them. Dementia will leave families sitting in silence. Lost for words. Having to relearn what it means to spend time with someone they've always known. This goes both ways. Living with dementia is a constant process of relearning for all affected. There are new moments again, and again, and again.

This book is about changing the story when it comes to dementia. For too long we have allowed fear of this disease to have the final say when it comes to defining personhood. Instead, the invitation is to talk about dementia in a new way; through the Way of unconditional Love and the bold presumption that we are never disconnected from each other.

Love is the unconditional source of all that unites us. It flows through, within, and between everything. Love transforms all our relationships, especially with those diagnosed with dementia. Some will call this Love God, but words are immaterial. In fact, with dementia we will eventually go beyond all words. The fruits of Love are joy and peace. These are the guiding lights in all we say and do. Love, joy, and peace guide us to go beyond the physical limitations of dementia into the unlimited capacity of all persons, no matter who they are, to positively affect, transform, and change lives. This is also how the world is changed. It might be hard to see this, but it is not difficult to experience. We just have to remain open-handed, non-judgemental, and curious especially when it comes to those we feel we have nothing in common. In this, Love is the great pretender. We are more connected to each other than we ever dreamed possible.

There is much lost with dementia and at the same time, there is an invitation to become immersed in a bigger story about ourselves and others. Through this story, we find that deep down we have the capacity to truly live in peace for the good of all. Those with dementia show us how to do this. They take us from the ordinary into the extraordinary. As such, you can be comforted with the knowledge that a loved One with dementia will continue to touch lives. They are our teachers and empower us with new insights into the human condition that will transform this world. See their light, for it does and will continue to shine brightly.

CASE STUDY: THE SILENT ONE SPEAKS

When I began visiting with Patty she was advanced in her dementia. She was entirely non-verbal and spent most of the day sleeping. She would sometimes be in her bed curled up tight like a little ball of twine. It was as if her whole body had turned inward and away from the world. She had little in the way of any ability to communicate. On a few occasions, she gave what might have been described as a half smile but otherwise, her demeanour was fixed.

One time I arrived to visit with Patty she was sitting in a wheelchair in the common area. It was a busy place and there was a lot of noise and activity, so I took her to a quieter area. I wanted to focus my full attention on her and being in a quieter place greatly assists with this. It also allows one to pick up on small sounds and body cues made by those who no longer communicate with words.

As Patty was a professing Christian, it felt appropriate to read Scripture with her. I read Psalm 23, a familiar source of comfort for the sick and dying. I also felt led to read these words from Psalm 103:

Praise God, my soul! Let all that is within me, praise God's holy name... Who redeems my life from destruction and crowns me with love and compassion.[2]

Reminding people that they wear a crown of Love invites them to affirm their personhood in a powerful way. We all wear this crown. Whatever anybody else has told us, whatever anyone has done to us, we are Loved. We are loved by God, and we are loved all the time. I also reminded Patty of the amazing things she had done in her life and played relaxing music to foster a peaceful and sacred environment. The entire time Patty gave me no indication she heard or understood anything said to her.

As the music played and I spoke with Patty, I held her hand and looked into her eyes. It felt like I was seeing her whole life before me; as if the books of her life were opened. Then, holding both her hands, I felt led to speak about how they had embraced her children, made things, cooked meals, and gifted a comforting and loving touch to many she had met. Her whole life was laid out beyond the limitations of her present physical form. This is also how God sees us. The lines on her face and hands became transformed into deep channels of Love etched into her body; a permanent reminder of the Loving smiles and gestures she had bequeathed to so many. There was such joy and peace as we sat together. She had spoken no words, but everything I felt she wanted to say had been heard.

As it came time to end the visit, I thanked God for Patty's life and this moment together. We had been on Holy ground and tears welled up in my eyes. Through her, I was gifted a powerful opportunity to see the way in which someone with dementia blesses lives. She was a remarkable person who had worked tirelessly in her lifetime, and now it was her time to rest. It was also her time to be served as she had served.

Connecting with the supreme source of Love will always take us beyond words and I pray that you will have the same experience of feeling this that I did with Patty. Because of her, I began this journey of understanding the power all persons have to truly impact the lives of others no matter who they are. The ripples of this moment continue to spread out across my life and the lives of others for all to see.

CASE STUDY: THE GIFT OF PRESENCE

Don was an educator who was in the middle of writing a book before life took a turn and he was diagnosed with dementia. The exact sequence of events I never learned, but when I met him he was in bed, wearing adult diapers, and barely able to speak. Whatever he did say was word salad. He drifted in and out of sleep during my visit with him.

As we saw with Patty, visiting those with dementia does not always involve having a conversation with them. Whilst we often want to talk with people, when it comes to dementia this can easily become frustrating and confusing especially when we ask them to remember things. We do not ask those with dementia to remember anything. Instead, we do the remembering for them. We are also there to provide companionship. Sometimes this can include talking with people, but it does not have to. We really want the One with dementia to feel Loved. People will remember how we made them feel.

During my visit with Don I sat next to him, held his hand, and played quiet music to foster a peaceful and sacred environment. Music truly is a universal language. A few times I talked about some things in his room to ascertain whether he remained connected to any of them. He was not. However, he did audibly respond to my speaking his daughter's name. He would also wake up each time I repositioned my hand, I guess thinking I was taking it away. Eventually, I needed to after sitting with him for almost an hour. He was peaceful and asleep when I left.

Afterwards, I called his daughter. Whilst my visit with Don had been an enjoyable experience, I began to hear how her visits with him were not so. She spoke of him becoming agitated while she was there, and not knowing what to talk about due to his incomprehensible speech. There was a great sense of lostness in her voice as she described this. She was grieving the loss of a deep connection they had once shared.

I do not know if she ever visited with Don after our phone call, but she did express appreciation for understanding how being present with someone with dementia is a gift; both for them and us. We explored various ways Don might have been seeking a deeper connection with her during their visits. For example, rather than seeing his agitation as Don not wanting her to be there, she welcomed the suggestion that it might have been him feeling frustrated that he could not communicate with her. His agitation was not a sign of wanting to be disconnected but more reconnected. We also spoke about how he had responded to her name and this too gave a sense of hope that he still knew and loved her. She began to see that visits with Don could consist of simply being present with him. He was inviting her to stay connected in new and deeper ways; beyond words. She went from being anxious to feeling hopeful.

Speaking with Don's daughter, I began to appreciate just how much the stories we tell ourselves affect the quality of our relationships. If we begin with a narrative of disconnection then we will seek and affirm the evidence for this. However, change the story to one of connection and our interactions become transformed. We connect to each other by being present and we are present when we are connected. The gift of presence is the story of connection.

17 EMPOWERING LIFE LESSONS

LESSON ONE:
LIFE IS SACRED

Dementia is the great leveller of life. It flattens the curve when it comes to gender, sexuality, notability, and achievement. Dementia doesn't care how much money you've got, what work you did, what house you lived in, what vacations you took, how many children you had, or whom you loved. This isn't to say none of this matters, but none of it matters now. When it comes to dementia we are all the same.

It is human nature to judge a person's worth by what they produce: what grades did you get, how much do you earn, and what do you do for work? We have been taught to ground our sense of self-worth in such things, but when it comes to dementia none of that matters. Instead, we are entirely person-centred.

To begin here is to put our life into a different context. It is the start of understanding what is truly important; a more simplified approach to living. Dementia takes many things away when it comes to memories and functionality and replaces these with childlike innocence. People are loved simply for being here; for their ongoing presence with us. In this, we think of a newborn baby. Babies come into the world unable to do anything for themselves and entirely dependent on others, but none of that takes anything away from the sacredness of their life. Babies are loved. That is all.

People want their life to have purpose and meaning, but this is not grounded in things they have done or will do. Functionality does not equal value. Our life has purpose and meaning simply because we are here. From the moment we were born to wherever we are at today, our life has made a difference. Our life impacts other lives. This world was unlike anything else prior to our birth, and it will be unlike anything else after we die. As such, our life has meaning and purpose for simply having been lived. We also have the opportunity to make a difference no matter who we are, so dwell in the joy of knowing that all lives matter.

LESSON TWO:
LIVE FOR THE MOMENT

Dementia leaves One living entirely in the moment. There is no past or future, just the Now. The person living with dementia does not wrestle with fears, doubts, or concerns about life. There are no temptations, procrastinating behaviours, or worries about what has been. Our loved One is not plagued by such things and if they are expressed, these are quickly dispelled by bringing them back into the moment. The Now.

With dementia, the mind is regularly purged and purified. Thoughts become ever simpler; each moment purer and purer as the disease progresses. The reality of the Now experienced by those with dementia is empowering. It is a place many seek to find through their spiritual practice; to be so utterly devoid of distracting thoughts and entirely centred in the Now. The One with dementia shows this is possible. In this, they have become spiritual Masters.

Oh that our minds were clear of all the thoughts holding us back. Oh, that we would truly understand the fragility of this life and simply get on with the task of living it. Too many opportunities have come and gone because we have talked ourselves out of them. A sense of call to do something or to become someone has been resisted due to living in fear of what others might think; worried about whether we have the skills or capacity to do it. For the One with dementia, there are no such concerns just the simplicity of the moment. The Now. They are who they are and they will be who they will be. I am, who I am.

The One with dementia also teaches us to let go. They show us that letting go of the past is possible and that we do not need to fear the future. Our minds can be purged of such things. Negative thoughts can be here one moment, and gone the next. So name them, accept they are here, and then let them go. Let them be here for the briefest of moments before becoming consumed by the unlimited potential you have to be your true self. Live for the moment in love, joy, and peace!

LESSON THREE:
LIVE YOUR TRUTH

It is a refreshing experience to spend time with someone and know you are able to be yourself. Whomever you are and whatever you believe, they don't judge you. They accept you no matter your religion, politics, gender, or sexuality. None of that is important. We get to show up just as we are. With such people, our world is also stripped bare of the many things others have used to divide us. There is no more us/them; either/or. It is simply we. WE are all welcome.

This basic acceptance of others is exemplified in the life of One with dementia. For them, everyone is a new friend and through them, we are transformed into a new state of being together. They show us that divisions can and will be overcome. With them, peace becomes the norm rather than the exception. They are prophets for our time and reveal the capacity we have to truly live in a different world. They empower us with a new vision of things to come; a new earth. If only we would lay aside all that we allow to divide us as they do. Wars and conflicts would cease.

To live with such openness is also a gift to others. Many wrestle with questions of purpose and personhood because they fear other people's reactions. Who we are and how we want to live can often become limited by worrying about this, rather than authentically living our core truth. With such a state of things, we are restless and lack peace. Being unsettled on the inside leads to unrest in the outside world. When people are not living in peace with who they are they will act out, vent their emotions, and harm those who seek to convince them otherwise. A person's greatest enemy will be the person they fear becoming.

So set your heart and mind to be empowered and impassioned by the Spirit of love, joy, and peace. Love who you are and love others for who they are. Celebrate all lives as the One with dementia does. Come together in joy and peace for the good of all. When we do this we will all get to enjoy the abundant fruits of life, liberty, and freedom.

LESSON FOUR:
TAKE TIME FOR OTHERS

Those living with dementia are truth-tellers. They tell you exactly how it is. They might not use normal modes of expression, but if they like you, you'll know it and if they don't, you'll know about that too. They won't beat about the bush. There's no passive-aggressiveness. They say what they say and that's that; deal with it.

Engaging with those living with dementia requires patience, empathy, and compassion. We know what they say comes wrapped up in their illness. At times they will steamroll over our emotions and when they do they don't apologise because they don't know they're doing it. Instead, we have to keep in mind that in another time and space they might not have said those things. We know there is more going on here. Their emotions pour into words that would have never been spoken.

Let's take this same experience and use it to pause in our interactions with each other, especially when critical words are spoken. Did they mean what they said? Are we the ones they are angry and irritated with? It's worth taking time to pause and detach ourselves from the negative emotions that arise; emotions that can be anger-fuelled and vengeful.

People with dementia invite us into an empowering silence. They create opportunities for us to learn to control and regulate our emotions and responses. When we find ourselves confused, upset, or hurt by something they said, another part of us is reminded that we are dealing with someone who has an illness impairing their thought process. This momentary pause is an empathic response. There is more going on.

How transformed the world would be if we took time to do this with all people. To not immediately react to something someone says or does, but to ask the question, "What's really going on?" Is this about me, or them? Did they really mean to say that, or are they trying to say something else? In some cases, a momentary pause and questions like this might literally become the difference between life and death.

LESSON FIVE:
TELL STORIES

We tell the ones with dementia stories about their life. We show them photos, watch videos, read books, and talk. We remind them of things they have done, places they have been, experiences they have had, and people they have forgotten. The aim of telling these stories is to help them reconnect with the life they have lived. We do not ask them to remember their life because they most likely do not. Instead, we do the remembering for them. Storytelling is also a very selective process. We tell stories that emotionally connect with them; the most fun and vibrant ones. In this, we remind them of their best life.

Sometimes people visiting with an abusive parent/partner will spend time trying to help them connect with a new story; one grounded in Love. Dementia has provided them with a blank canvas on which to paint a new picture of their life. They see their loved One in a deeper way. They know there is Good inside them, for they have seen glimpses of this throughout their life. Now they are given the opportunity to tell this story in full; a new story. To redeem a life. This is a supreme act of Love. Helping someone to remember all the Good they are too.

It is easy to get stuck just telling old stories; stories about others and also our own life. Stories grounded in anger, shame, and judgement. Yet when we introduce new stories we become empowered to live new lives. The stories we tell fundamentally shape and define the quality of all our relationships, both with others and also ourselves. If the story we tell is about being a bad person, we will live that story. If the story is about people never achieving their dreams, we will never try to achieve ours. However, change the story, decide to tell new stories, or even edit an old story to highlight the things we are truly capable of, and our lives will be transformed. The old will go and the new will come.

Also, if you love telling great stories about other people's lives, then be sure to always do that for your own life too.

LESSON SIX:
RECEIVE GOOD GIFTS

We do not know why some things in life happen, and why some things do not. The certainties of life lie in our birth and death. All who are born will die, and no one dies without having first been born. What happens between life and death is unknown; an empowering and freeing thought.

Being here to experience life is a gift. This is why life is precious and sacred. It is an incredible thing to be in this world and to see what life is all about. In this, we are explorers setting out into uncharted territories without a map. Instead, we create the map as we go through life. It emerges as we chart our journey and each one of them is unique. None of us will experience this life the same way as others. There will only ever be one of you living your own life.

For some, their journey will take them into the Way of dementia. They too are engaged in the process of unfolding life's deepest mysteries. We all are until the moment we die. As long as we have breath we will do this. Each moment is also an opportunity to grow in our spirit. We might not see it like that at first, but approaching life open-handed is really the only way we will transform pain into something beautiful.

Some moments in life will leave us frustrated, depressed, and angry. Dementia is one such moment. We could remain in this state, or we can choose to adopt a different approach. Either way, it is coming at you. Being a free receiver of the gift of life is really the only thing we can control. These difficult moments also teach us not to hold onto pain and use it to inflict injury on others. Instead, with time, patience, and practice we can find the joy and peace present in all life's moments, even the difficult ones. When we eventually do find them, we identify them as good gifts to pass on to others. Each moment in life is brimming with abundant opportunities to do this; to seek out the good things and pass them on. May we remain open-handed and curious to find and receive the good gifts life offers, for they are there, always.

LESSON SEVEN:
THE GIFT OF TIME

Time is something those with dementia appear to have in abundance. They have time for everyone and everything. They have time for rest, activity, and sitting quietly. They are not rushing to get anywhere, and they have no pressing need to be doing anything. For the most part, they live contended lives. Whilst time is typically understood in a linear fashion, for One living with dementia it is more of a series of loops. They do not perceive time as an ever-expanding accumulation of knowledge or experiences but just a series of moments they will often revisit. This is why it's important to stay in sync with them. Avoid frustrations and difficulties arising by trying to keep them in a linear understanding of time. They are not there anymore and can become upset if we try to make it seem as if they are, or are meant to be.

There is also the gift of a different quality of time together. For example, if someone took time each week to visit the nail salon, now they gift us the time and opportunity to do a manicure for them. We get to pamper them. This regifting of time fosters precious reconnection. Or maybe someone was always busy, out of the house, in a rush, and doing things. Maybe growing up, children did not get to spend as much time with a parent as they wanted, whereas now they can. There's no more rushing about, just time to be still and be together.

In this, we break open the narrative that attaches self-worth to our use of time. We are often deemed to be doing something worthwhile if we are using our time productively, or a useful person when doing something worthwhile. However, the One with dementia is under no such compulsion to be productive and instead, they are given the gift of time to simply be who they are. They live the truth of these words: I am who I am. Therefore, let us be empowered by their example. Take time to enjoy life and welcome all those who get to enjoy it with us. Also, take time to be still and rest. Being constantly busy is not always useful.

LESSON EIGHT:
THE RHYTHM OF LIFE

There is a time for everything. A time for work, and a time for rest. It is okay to rest. It is okay to be still and do nothing. It is okay to sleep. The One with dementia is our teacher when it comes to sleeping. With this, they empower us with a new story. They sleep whenever they feel the need to do so. Even whilst in our presence. They make few apologies for having fallen asleep. It is as natural to them as breathing.

Rest is something we were born to do. We let babies sleep because we know this is necessary for their health and growth. It is also necessary for those caring for them to get some much-needed respite. For careers of those with dementia, it is vitally important that they take time to rest. They MUST rest. To let someone rest is a loving thing to do.

When it comes to our physical needs, we have to pay attention to the rhythm of our bodies. Our body exerts energy and becomes tired. It will let us know when rest is needed and we are wise to pay attention to this. We cannot expect to power on through the days without this taking some physical toll on us. Those denied proper rest will soon become irritable, experience health concerns, and eventually burn out. The same is true when it comes to refreshing our whole being; our spiritual self. Take time to disconnect from the demands of the day and be still. Rest, reset, and recentre yourself. Some will do this by taking a nap, others by taking a walk, whilst others with prayer and meditation. In whatever capacity it is right for you to do this, set aside some time during the day to be still. This is not only necessary for our health but it is also something that will bring us joy and peace.

The One with dementia also teaches us the rhythm of words. We might not comprehend all someone is saying but sounds still have a flow to them. Match this and their tone. Like a band playing together, maintain tempo and harmony. Let your words sing to lift their mood. Also, have fun, play Jazz, improvise, and repeat the chorus over and over.

LESSON NINE:
RESET YOUR RELATIONSHIPS

To say to someone, "I forgive you" is an empowering thing. It is a relief to be forgiven for misdeeds, for misspoken words, for things we did to hurt others, and for things others have done to hurt us; to hold no grudges and reset our relationships. This is peacemaking behaviour and it truly transforms the world.

We are empowered by the life of the One with dementia to live this way. For them, every moment is a new moment. They welcome their friends as friends and their enemies as friends. With them, divisions are overcome. All are welcome. How do they do this? They dwell in the presence of unconditional love, for Love keeps no record of wrongs.

The potential for people to be in a different mode of relationship with each other is seen in the life of One with dementia. They show us that when the ability to hold a grudge and remain angry with someone is taken away, people's lives reset to the default of Love. Love is our *modus operandi*; our true state of being. We hate others and remain angry with them out of choice. Grudges are held onto with intention, and they are released the same way (intentionally).

Sometimes the One with dementia exhibits angry behaviours. These are normal human feelings. For some, being angry is a stage in their disease progression but they will not remain like this forever. No one is angry all the time. Eventually, the storm will pass. Peace will come. We forgive others in the knowledge that anger does represent their true self.

Let us, therefore, strive to live in peace with each other, for this really is possible as our experience serving those with dementia shows. With them, we are given an opportunity to turn unhealthy emotional responses into positive ones. They gift us the opportunity to practice restraint and redirection. Through this, we learn to promote peace; to be peacemakers. If we can do this with those living with dementia, then we can do it for all. Reset your relationships for the good of all.

LESSON TEN:
I AM BECAUSE WE ARE

There is so much we rely on from others. Just the simple act of eating anything involves a chain of multiple entities, behind which are numerous individuals working. In African philosophy, the concept of *Ubuntu* describes this mode of interconnectedness: I am because we are. Whilst there will always be things we can do for ourselves, when we meditate on just how much others do for us it shines a light on exactly how much we need each other; how together we truly are.

As dementia progresses a person's mobility and functionality are impacted and they become dependent on others for their activities of daily living (ADLs). When someone's dementia is defined as severe, they will require total assistance with all ADLs. Left alone in this state, they would soon die.

Truth is, very few of us would survive for very long in this world without the full and invested care of others. Our basic needs for clean water, food, clothing, energy, and fuel depend entirely on the work others do on our behalf. Therefore, let us live in gratitude for the work these Wonderful Ones do to ensure our own ADLs are met.

Being grateful for the work others do is also an invitation to live in peace with them. Lest we imagine this to be overly Idealistic, let's draw once again from the well of experience when serving those with dementia. Their natural state is one of Love, the fruits of which are joy and peace and they experience this when we are patient, kind, and protective of them. These basic ADLs are normal for everyone.

Ultimately, we create the conditions that lead people to want to take care of us by how we treat others. We are called to leave people better off than we find them. In this, we are empowered and inspired by how we care for our Beloved Ones with dementia. Our caring for them helps us see and experience our unlimited capacity to do Good to all persons, no matter who they are, for the good of all.

LESSON ELEVEN:
WORLD SOUL

Music is an indisputable connector of people. The differences between us become inconsequential when listening to and playing music. Go anywhere you find music being played, and you will find people across the spectrum of human expression listening to it. People of all varieties enjoy the same music. Rhythm unites people across gender, sexuality, economic status, legal status, culture, and even cognitive ability. It is a universal language. It will soothe, woo, and excite people everywhere.

A song can transport us into the past and emotionally transform us in the present. No matter how much someone declines cognitively, a tune will always find its way inside them. There is something familiar in music. Even when someone's speech is no longer coherent they will communicate with us via the rhythm, sound, and intonation of their words. These are the things that touch us. That we can still connect with One with dementia in this way shows just how deep the capacity for connection is. On the surface we might appear disconnected, but underneath, where the rhythm flows, we are a united people.

Once again we see that when our mind is stripped bare of resistance we are in a place of openness and acceptance. This is not to say that any words we speak, or any music we play, are going to resonate well with all people but that the capacity for connecting is always there. Seek to maximise this connection. Sometimes playing music might lead to unexpected sounds being heard unexpectedly, but we will always know when we are playing the right song (or speaking the right words) because the fruits of love, joy, and peace are present. The right words and music will elicit this response from even the most advanced in their dementia and shows just how possible it is to connect deeply with people in this Way. So let's draw from this truth about the human condition and use it to write new songs about our life together. Let's teach the world to sing in perfect harmony!

LESSON TWELVE:
IN THE COMPANY OF ANGELS

We are surrounded by angelic beings. In this world and the one that lies beyond, there are spiritual beings who support us as we journey through life. This is most evident as one approaches death. Working in hospice, we have been with many who in their final moments have experienced visions of what lies beyond or had visits from those who have passed before them. Whatever these experiences are, they invite us to take comfort in the knowledge that we are not alone.

We want people to experience a good death. In many respects, death is about birthing people from this life into the next. The experience of death shares many features in common with giving birth in this world. One of the clearest examples is when the breathing of the dying becomes heavy and panting, a sound reminiscent of a woman's breath pattern when having contractions and giving birth.

Death is the ultimate moment of birthing from this world, but the One with dementia has been on this journey long before this happens. Their release from this life began as their memory declined and with this, they experience a greater spiritual connection to all. In many respects, they become like angels; those who exist in a perfect state of being between this world and the next. Dementia also turns them inwards, toward their inner light, as cognitive, emotional, and spiritual experiences are freed from worldly distractions.

Angels are also strangers we befriend in this life. They lift people up. Those who care for loved Ones with dementia are angels who come alongside families in their time of need. When they transfer, turn, and move the sick and dying they are literally Angels of Mercy.

When all is said and done, angels bring peace. They invite us to not live in fear: "Be not afraid." Like them, we are called to help people find peace throughout their whole life, not just at the time of death. This is in fact our highest calling. May we be those who live accordingly.

LESSON THIRTEEN:
OUR RELIGIOUS IMAGINATION

Those living with dementia empower us to tell new stories about God. Over time, as they gradually forget old stories, they make room for new ones. This is particularly important for people to do when it comes to religious beliefs. Some people need to hear a different story when it comes to their religion, especially when beliefs have been grounded in guilt, shame, and judgement. We were not given the gift of life just to feel guilty about it, or be told over and over again that we will never be good enough. If this has been your experience, it's time for a change!

When it comes to the story of God in our life, each of us is on our own unique journey. We are not all the same and we will not experience God the same way. It is to be expected that people will have different beliefs from each other. We also do not need to concern ourselves with the form of religious practice or the matter of true religion. None of this troubles the One with dementia, just the fruit. It is our duty to ensure people are rooted in the fruits of love, joy, and peace when it comes to their faith. To do this, we always ground their story in God's unconditional Love.

As people with dementia approach the end of their life, we invite them into the greatest story we can tell about the value of their life here, as well as the place they will go to next. This life is not an accident. Their life has had a purpose. They will also go to a Loving place of peace. If they are not able to tell these stories for themselves, we will do it for them. Their story must be one where tears of sorrow are no more, and where mourning, crying, and pain have ceased. The old ways must pass.

In this, we affirm our intrinsic connectedness to the Divine source of Love. This is the Love that has shaped all lives. It is the Ground of our Being. If Love were not here, nothing else would be here, for love does not delight in the evil that destroys. With Love, we also offer people forgiveness and hope of eternal rest. Let nothing remain between us, them, and God. Ensure all are ready to depart.

LESSON FOURTEEN:
WHERE YOU GO I WILL GO

Dementia is a disease where people will go to a place others cannot follow. Our commitment is that whilst they will eventually leave us, we will not leave them. This is also our greatest gift to them. Most people die alone, but they do not want to die lonely.

Being united with others includes many things, mostly our direct presence with them, but it particularly involves our spirit. We can be in the presence of someone and not feel united with them. We are distant from them, as they are to us. Divisions occur when we allow someone or something to come between us. Certain words may have been spoken and pains endured. This is when the One with dementia leads us in the Way of grace and peace. They show us that it is possible to let things go. Over time, nothing will keep us from them. They will forget who their enemy is and welcome all. The old ways will eventually go. Forgiving and forgetting are also the Way of God.

As the One with dementia journeys into the peace that passes all understanding, we remain with them and reap the fruit of their Spirit. They bless and refresh us. This is their gift of bringing heaven to earth. This is also an invitation to become divided from all that brings a lack of peace in the world; to be zealous and passionate for peace. To let peace come and not resist this. The One with dementia shows us that it is possible to let peace come.

When we insist on people doing it our way we foster divisions, and if they do not come with us we're stuck. Divided. Instead, the righteous middle way is to come together. To find the common middle ground. We see this in the life of the One with dementia as they become increasingly open to our leading them; taking care of them. They also lead us. In time, all resistance will be overcome. We are drawn to them, and they are drawn to us. We journey together. Meeting in the middle. Holding each other close. Letting nothing come between us for the Good of all.

LESSON FIFTEEN:
LOVE

So many people in this world are desperate to feel and experience Love. So many people are hurting. So much suffering. Our care for those who are the least among us empowers the world with a new vision of what it means to truly Love others. To be devoted to one another. Crave this Love. We desperately need to experience this Love.

So much is allowed to come between us and all for nothing. In the end, none of it matters. Your life and this world will pass away. The things we deem important will one day become unimportant. It will all be gone. We hold out hope that one day this world will be a better place, in the future, but we have the potential for that to happen in our lifetime right now. We just have to become like the One with dementia who forgives all our misdeeds and remembers them no more. In this, the least among us are leading the Way. They show the world what is truly possible.

Those diagnosed with dementia have also gifted us the opportunity to become vessels of Love for them; conduits of unconditional Love. Through them, our lives are immersed in the transforming presence of Love. This is also God's Love. Holding nothing back. Welcoming all and receiving all. Together, we experience this Love. We are empowered by a new Spirit through which the earth is transformed. Whilst we are so easily lost in our own thoughts, we can be readily found again. We have the capacity to do this. Don't let anyone convince you otherwise. In fact, we show we have found Love, and our minds are transformed, when we serve the One with dementia and witness the ever-present capacity for doing Good to others. Our servant heart.

So remain open to this Way. Allow your whole life to be transformed by the fullness of God's abiding Love. Nothing can or will ever separate you from it. Nothing! Believe it! Your life and that of your Loved Ones are precious and sacred. Let no one convince you otherwise. Don't let anyone deny you the right and the opportunity to live in God's Love.

LESSON SIXTEEN:
BEYOND THE PHYSICAL

"Luminous beings are we, not this crude matter"[3]

With dementia, it is easy to focus on just the losses. These are felt, experienced and tangible. At the same time, dementia is one of many types of disease people will die from. Someone has not been dealt a bad hand in life (or punished by God) because they have dementia. You could die from any one of a number of diseases. That said, dementia is a special kind of ailment that takes people on a unique journey.

In this book, those diagnosed with dementia are spoken of in a powerful and empowering way. They are more than broken bodies. They are those whose light is shining brightly. When we operate with a narrative of usefulness, people with dementia will be deemed no longer useful and left in the dark. Expectations will not be met. People will be disappointed. That's why we uncover their light. We reveal it and see them from a new perspective; through a different lens. When we do this, their inner light shines brightly. They illuminate OUR Way.

It is possible to speak about life in just material terms. Life is what it is. Random. A cosmic accident. We are here because we could be and we remain here simply because we can. However, the One with dementia invites us into a bigger story. They draw us into a liminal space where there is a deeper meaning and purpose to all this.

How they do this is in the Way they take us beyond the physical. We get to see the world and our life differently through them. They have also shaped our being here long before we arrived, and they will continue to do that long after they die. We owe our very humanity to them. For what elevates us above other species is the will and capacity to care for the least among us. They showed us how to do this through their care of us, and now we get to do it for them. This is also God's work in us. We return to dust, but we are at the same time much more than this.

LESSON SEVENTEEN:
INVITATION

This is a book about empowerment. It is also a book about hope. It is about seeing greatness in people. ALL people. When we are consumed by disempowering stories we are kept from living our best life with others. Change the story and everything in the world will change.

Dementia is not a contagious disease. However, we want our efforts to promote a better world to be just that. Contagious Love. Contagious joy. Contagious peace. All this is grounded in unconditional Love. One example of what this Love looks like is seen in how we care for those with dementia. Love is patient, kind, and forgiving of them. This is also the work of peacemaking that creates new worlds.

So many are keeping things locked up tight inside that are preventing them from having a relationship with others, but when the capacity to remember these things is no longer there life becomes different. We live in freedom and become open to a new Way. With dementia, we get to see just how quickly this can happen. Forgiveness in a matter of moments; in the blink of an eye. People forget the things keeping them apart from others and live in a new way. Letting go of the old and embracing the new. So let's do that while we are able to actively participate in this. Don't wait until the choice is no longer ours to make. There are moments when life shows us that even in the most difficult of circumstances, divisions can and will be overcome. Peace will reign.

This fruit is also the work of God. With God, it is always about being fruitful. Opening things up. Enlarging borders. When God does prune, this is to bring more fruit elsewhere. God is also the great recycler. With God, nothing is wasted. So immerse your life into a story of God that fully and unconditionally accepts all you are. You are not the sum of the worst things you have done, nor the worst things that have happened to you. You are a luminous being whose light shines brighter than you can possibly imagine. See your light. You are amazing. We all are!

FAST SCORES

Dementia is ageing backwards. The trajectory of the disease is one where people literally go from functioning adulthood into a dependent and infantile state. This is not a derogatory assessment but the reality of where people typically end up. To help understand and determine the stages someone is at in their dementia, the Functional Assessment Staging Tool (FAST) is a clinical tool used to plot declines as the disease progresses. The language of FAST is specifically designed for clinicians to chart declines. However, when we focus on just the declines it will lead us to see dementia more in terms of loss, and this can become a significant source of grief as families and loved Ones navigate the changes. It also overlooks the fact that loss is not all there is. A more inclusive understanding of the FAST system, such as the one proposed here, is an invitation to explore life in deeper ways. It will empower people to transform all their relationships.

A diagnosis of dementia does not need to stop people in their tracks but can invite them to navigate their relationships with others in new ways; to fully enjoy their time together. May you always dwell in the joy of simply being here with your loved Ones, no matter where they are in their journey of life.

ALPHA

FAST score 2: Subjective functional deficit

Let's begin by noting how common it is for people to experience memory decline as they age. We all forget things at times and FAST score 2 describes this typical experience. When we do forget something it also takes nothing away from who we are. We are still the same person, just someone who forgot something. This is even true when it comes to losing a limb. We don't see someone as anything less than the person they were when they had all their limbs intact, although we also cannot deny that their life has changed and they will need some different accommodations now. The same is true when we hear about dementia. It would not be fair or accurate to regard someone diagnosed with this disease as anything less than the person they have always been. Of course, they too will need different accommodations as things change for them, but when it comes to who they are in their core being nothing has been lost. It is all still there, albeit in an increasingly inaccessible form as they journey with this disease.

BETA

FAST score 3: Objective functional deficit interferes with a person's most complex task - Mental age: 12+ years

Dementia becomes a medical diagnosis when it impacts a person's life in such a way that it leaves them vulnerable. FAST score 3 identifies the beginning of this journey and the difficulties someone is starting to have doing things such as going to new places and organising themselves. This is particularly noticeable when routines are broken. It is also something becoming increasingly evident to others. Cognitively, someone at this stage is said to be in a teen phase. This is not to disparage teenagers but to note how in hindsight we had much to learn in this phase of life. If we think of dementia as a gradual unlearning of things, we can begin to see that someone in this stage is starting to lose touch with things they have learned to do. They are ageing backwards. Complicated things are becoming harder to do. Life is getting confusing.

In their teenage years, people struggle with understanding who they are, especially as their bodies change. The same is true of One with dementia. They need us to be patient, compassionate, and supportive as things change for them. In the teen years, there is also a willingness to experiment and try new things. People get curious. So when we think of the One with dementia in this stage of life, rather than keep reminding them of things they used to do, or become frustrated when they are not able to do them, we might instead wonder what new things they are becoming open to. Spiritually, they might be receptive to new beliefs and ideas. Personally, we can find them open to healing broken relationships and welcoming people into their life in a new way.

GAMMA

FAST score 4: Instructional Activities of Daily Living (IDLs) become affected, such as bill paying, cooking, cleaning, travelling - Mental age: 8-12 years

Those in this stage of dementia are said to experience the world the same way 8-year-olds do, with a FAST score of 4 describing how life is becoming more streamlined for them. Simple things they once did have started to become difficult to do without assistance. In fact, one thing dementia will eventually bring is freedom from all the things we spend our lives worrying and stressing about such as bills, what to wear, cooking, cleaning, etc. That's not to say people in this stage of life are giving up, not at all, they are just on a unique journey to greater freedom. People are also still very mobile so there are many ways to help them live life to the full such as going on trips or even vacations. Just be flexible, don't plan too much, and provide lots of opportunities for downtime. In fact, the goal is for all our lives to be relaxed and free of stress and worry; the way many kids experience things. So go for it, and have fun!!!

DELTA

FAST score 5: Needs help selecting proper attire - Mental age: 5-7 years

Between the ages of 5-7, children are starting to become more independent. Yet with dementia, and as people age backwards, FAST score 5 describes the increasing need to depend on others, especially for activities of daily living (ADLs). A loved One will need help with lots of different things, such as toileting, making sure they don't fall and bump into things, making sure they are eating well, taking care of their appearance, bathing, and simply getting about.

Emotions may also be tricky to navigate at this stage, so we are gifted the opportunity to practice a lot of patience with them. With this comes the opportunity to talk, play, and in particular tell incredible stories. In fact, this can be a richly creative time as people take us on some amazing journeys through their life. Some of these will be grounded in reality, and some will be drawn from their imagination. That's okay, for in many ways we enter a more dreamlike phase with them. Speech becomes fluid. Reality blurs. Sometimes people will be telling us familiar things in a different way or in a new way. Words are not always used in direct association and can become more expressive of feelings and emotions. This is something we all do. This is also why we use our words carefully so as not to hurt others and if we do, we will learn through our care of One with dementia to speak healing words in response.

EPSILON

FAST score 6a: Needs help putting on clothes - Mental age: 5 years

When someone is assessed with a FAST score of 6a they are defined as "Moderately Severe" in their dementia. People are more dependent on others for their ADLs. Speech is becoming limited. In time, independent behaviours and verbal responses will be reduced to nil.

People at this stage are operating with the mental capacity of a 5-year-old. Being a 5-year-old is not without its emotional challenges, and this is also true for One with dementia. Some of this will be caused by them sensing something is not quite right and becoming frustrated at not fully comprehending what this is. This is why we will at times metaphorically dress them in the clothing of a 5-year-old as this will assist us with remembering they are no longer functioning at a level we have always known and expected them to. We also celebrate the young amongst us. They are fun and enjoyable to be around. They also need their clothing to be loose. They like to be free. Comfort is most important at this stage so they can play and be themselves. The same is true of One with dementia. Let them be free to wear what they want and if they make a mess, things can be easily washed.

ZETA

With FAST score 6b, we are moving into the realm of helping someone take care of their personal and intimate ADLs. This begins with bathing, but it will soon include other needs. Sometimes these needs will overlap with others, but we must keep in mind that a person with dementia will never go backwards in the FAST system. If they are diagnosed FAST 6c one week, they will not be diagnosed 6b the next. Dementia is a degenerative disease.

When it comes to bathing, this is a very private thing and people have very individualised habits around self-care. To let someone else bathe us is also especially intimate, both for the one being cared for and for family members who may have employed someone to do this. Here we draw inspiration from the One with dementia, for their life becomes ever more open to trusting others. In this, they call us to be trusting and trustworthy. They show that even when we are at our most vulnerable, there are many ready and willing to support and care for us. Whilst dementia seems to be a lonely experience, we are more deeply connected to each other than it might first appear.

ETA

FAST score 6c: Needs help toileting - Mental age: 4 years

With FAST score 6c we continue to acknowledge a decline away from independence towards dependence as the One with dementia is now assisted with their toileting needs. At the same time, it is another way life is becoming ever more simplified for them; one less thing to worry about.

When we help someone with their toileting needs we hold them in the highest esteem, for this is the way royalty has been treated across the ages. Kings and queens regularly employed someone to assist them with their toileting needs, especially when this was difficult for them. This means both the great and those regarded as the least amongst us have required assistance in these personal matters. We also remember that God crowns each one of us with Love and compassion. In this, we are all Kings and Queens together.

Young children also need help with their toileting needs, and often on the potty kids love to hear stories. So tell your Loved Ones stories of how much they are unconditionally Loved. Tell everyone in the world this story, especially the One with dementia. Also, sing to them, play with them, and read simple books with lots of pictures; anything to keep us connected and to celebrate all we are.

THETA

FAST score 6d: Urinary incontinence - Mental age: 3-4 years

For too long shame has been associated with dementia, especially when it comes to incontinence. Why is that? This is a disease, so let's change that story. People are not choosing to get dementia and become incontinent. It just happens. We would not think of shaming someone for getting cancer and their body losing functionality, so let's stop doing that when it comes to dementia. As this disease progresses, incontinence will happen.

FAST score 6d identifies this unique point. It is another sign that someone is moving closer to the end. Yet whilst they have breath in their lungs and their body is functioning normally - yes, pooping and peeing are normal bodily functions - we get to celebrate their continued presence with us. We also do this for our little Ones when they potty train. We encourage and support them with words such as: "No problem! Accidents happen! Let's get you cleaned up and changed." No shame, no judgment, just reassurance, support, and Love. Always Love!

IOTA

FAST score 6e: Fecal incontinence - Mental age: 2-3 years

The presence of fecal matter is both natural and a significant source of contention for humans. Humans poop, we all do, but unlike urine, this requires some effort when it comes to cleaning up. We can't really poop and go! Also, poop has negative connotations associated with it. For example, we will talk about someone having almost peed themselves with laughter as a positive thing (comedy-induced incontinence), but tell some to clean up their crap as indicative of a problem.

With FAST 6e, we also arrive at the final stage in someone's journey from moderately severe dementia (FAST 6a-e) to severe dementia (FAST 7a-f). Yet as with all the stages, this is not a qualitative journey but a quantitive one. For to suggest that FAST 6e is any worse or better than any of the other stages is incorrect. It just is. It is one in a series of moments in someone's journey with dementia. It also means that any need to be taken to the bathroom has now been eliminated and along with that the potential for falls. Anxiety and fear are reduced. So whilst we might not necessarily enjoy dealing with the fallout from someone pooping and peeing, things have become more relaxed with them.

TAU

FAST score 7a: Speaks 5-6 words during the day -
Mental age:18 months

With FAST 7a, we enter the stage of dementia known as "Severe." Language has become reduced to a series of limited verbal responses throughout the day. The body is slowly shutting down. The One with dementia is turning inward and away from the world. They will sleep more. There is very little need and desire for communication with words. Instead, this is done through presence, touch, and trial and error. We can liken this to learning the needs, wants, and desires of children aged between 12-18 months. Typically, those assessed at FAST 7 have a life expectancy of 12-18 months. We are now in the final stages of this disease before death comes.

Fewer words are not just a sign that someone is dying. They also indicate that one is closer to God. Often we define someone's relationship with God according to the words they use, but the truth is human language will never fully grasp and comprehend God's infinite reality. The spiritually wise affirm the presence of God with silence. With God, less is more. With this in mind, the One with dementia challenges us to go beyond the surface to connect with what truly unites us. Words divide. Knowledge puffs up. Love builds up. Love will always unite. Become still and know God and others in the presence of Love.

UPSILON

FAST score 7b: Speaks only 1 word clearly - Mental age:12 months

With FAST 7b, the One with dementia is moving into pure presence. As the wise Ones have taught us, our being here in the world is an opportunity to serve each other in Love. This is our true call; our Divine calling. The One with dementia allows us to fulfill this in a unique way. Life is not an accident. All have the purpose to unite with others for the Good of all.

Talking to the One with dementia about their life will immerse them into our story of their life, but the truth of this life as they have known it is now beyond our understanding. It always was. They have held many things back; words from being spoken and things from being done. They will carry secrets to the grave. They have also saved many from the hurt and pain of harsh words and deeds. This is Love. The ultimate act of Love is to hold back anything that will cause harm to others. We do not want to add trouble to the world. Instead, we Love and celebrate those whose presence allows us to sing to them, massage them, brush their hair, hold their hand, and wrap them in blankets. We do this for them; we do it for all. Treating others with the respect and dignity we want others to show us. For one day, we too will become the One in need.

PHI

FAST score 7c: Can no longer walk - Mental age:12 months

With FAST 7c, the One with dementia stops walking. They continue to move in other ways, but no longer this way. Their time to be still has come. It is the Sabbath their body was aching for. Weary legs and knees are resting. How many miles those legs and knees have walked and run is beyond counting. All we know is that there will be no more walking. The time to get off the beaten path has arrived.

When people are incapable of walking they will be carried. To be carried is not just a sign of need but also status. We lift up those who have achieved great things among us. We also lift up symbols of greatness such as trophies and holy artifacts. Not just anyone gets to lift these great things up, just those uniquely set aside for the task. As such, when people are appointed to lift up the One with dementia it is a recognition of the trust being placed in them to do this. It is also an acknowledgment of their special status in society. Honour is being doubly bestowed; on the One being lifted up and on those tasked to do this. It is an honourable thing to be carried by others as much as it is to be asked to carry them.

CHI

FAST score 7d: Can no longer sit up - Mental age:6-9 months

FAST 7d is the point at which the One with dementia has lost the ability to remain upright. They also spend more time lying down. Sleeping. Ageing backwards will lead someone to this point. It is a natural progression of things and one that will eventually end with them going to sleep forever.

Their laying down has also occurred as they have given up things and sacrificed their own wants and needs for the sake of others. Through this, they laid down their whole life. Many times they have put to death their own needs and wants. Being no longer able to sit up has also flattened their body; their face turned towards the world they have known whilst their back is pressed towards the ground where they will soon return. They remind us that all return to the dust from which we came. Life is always lived in the shadow of death, but we must not fear this. Instead, we are invited to live in such a manner that we are able to sleep peacefully; to not act in ways that prevent ourselves or others from enjoying peaceful sleep at night. For whenever we sleep we rest in the presence of Divine Love.

PSI

FAST score 7e: Can no longer smile - Mental age:2-4 months

When we are smiling we are emotionally connected to someone or something. Smiling is a moment of recognition. With FAST 7e, the One with dementia is no longer connected to the world and others in this way. Instead, their face is turned toward the world to come as they understand this to be. Most of us do not know what the world to come will be like. A few have had glimpses, but only those who have passed over have attained the fullness of this knowledge. For the rest of us, we are left to ponder the great beyond. Staring into the thin space between life and death. Seeking to understand what lies beyond.

The One with dementia teaches us not to fear what lies ahead. For their journey has ended in a place of contemplation; a place of stillness and preparation. They show us that when our heart is at peace, when everything has been stripped away and life becomes a series of simple moments, there really is nothing to fear. In this, they are like newborns who do know what lies ahead in this life but sense they are in a Loving presence. They trust that they are safe; that their needs will be met. They also do not arrive in the world smiling, but one day they will. One day they will smile at the One who has loved them from the beginning. The One who has always been there. For whilst they know in part now, one day they will see face to face. We all will.

43

OMEGA

FAST score 7f: Can no longer hold up head - Mental age:0-2 months

With FAST 7f, the One with dementia takes their final bow and bids adieu. Their life commended to others and God as they understand God to be. Naked they came into the world and naked they depart from it. All they have been and all they have done wrapped into these final moments. A life lived. Complete.

We celebrate the One who has journeyed with us, brought us into the world, and kept us in it. Their life folded into ours. They will go on living within us, through us, and eternally in the world and beyond. Bow towards them in honour and celebration for all the Good they are. Grief will also lower our heads and drops us to our knees. Through our tears, we will sing their praises. We bless them for their Holy presence in our life; my alpha, in your omega.

Stage Name	FAST score	Empowering characteristics of the One with dementia	Mental age
ALPHA	2	Memory decline as a common experience	-
BETA	3	Curious and open to new things	12+ years
GAMMA	4	Free of stress and worry	8-12 years
DELTA	5	Imaginative and creative	5-7 years
EPSILON	6a	Letting the inner child emerge	5 years
ZETA	6b	Trusting of others	4 years
ETA	6c	Loving and feeling loved	4 years
THETA	6d	Being yourself	3-4 years
IOTA	6e	Living without fear and anxiety	2-3 years
TAU	7a	Rest, sleep, silence	18 months
UPSILON	7b	Letting go of the past	12 months
PHI	7c	Lifting others up	12 months
CHI	7d	Laying down our life for the sake of others	6-9 months
PSI	7e	Turning away from this world	2-4 months
OMEGA	7f	Adieu	0-2 months

SHINY MOMENTS

Use the following pages to record empowering moments of learning and special times of connection with your Wonderful One.

They are a light to guide your Way.

NOTES

[1] All names have been changed

[2] Adapted from Psalm 103: 1, 4

[3] Yoda, Star Wars: Episode V - The Empire Strikes Back

Printed in Great Britain
by Amazon